No Gym Required: A Guide to Losing Weight From Home - 50 Easy Workouts From Home, 30 Day No Gym Routine Included!

Jim Murillo

Everyone has a dream body they wish to achieve, this book is written to help you get just that.

Free time is becoming rarer and rarer as the years go by, with the average American citizen working 40 hours per week, time is hard to come by, meaning a lot of people are neglecting their body by not commuting to a gym. This is where this book comes in. In this book you will find 50 easy, simple to use workouts that require no gym equipment, as well as a 30-day routine designed for people who lead busy lives and don't have the time it takes commute to a gym and workout for 2 hours every single day. Every workout in this book can be done at home as you don't require any special equipment. The workouts are divided into 5 sections, Full body, Legs, Shoulders and Arms, Core, Chest and Back so you know what muscles each workout targets. Using the knowledge you've gained from this book you can make your own workout routine that suits your lifestyle and goals, or you can use the 30 day routine provided in the book.

I have been working out using these methods for the past 10 years and have seen enormous change in body despite being a full-time dad, working a full-time computer engineering job, all while learning becoming a certified personal trainer. Now my job is to help hard working people become fit and achieve their dream body.

It has been proven that regular exercise not only contributes to a healthier, longer life, but it also helps greatly with mental health. The mere act of exercising can help reduce stress, anxiety and give you a more positive outlook on life.

I am not joking when I say staying fit is the number one most important thing you can do for yourself in order to improve your life. These workouts will not only change your life, it will make you happier, healthier and allow you take make the most of your time on Earth.

Contents

Full Body Workouts

Plank

Lie down with your face looking at the floor, make an L shape with your arms with your forearms on the floor and hands clasped. Straighten your back and tighten your abs. Hold this position.

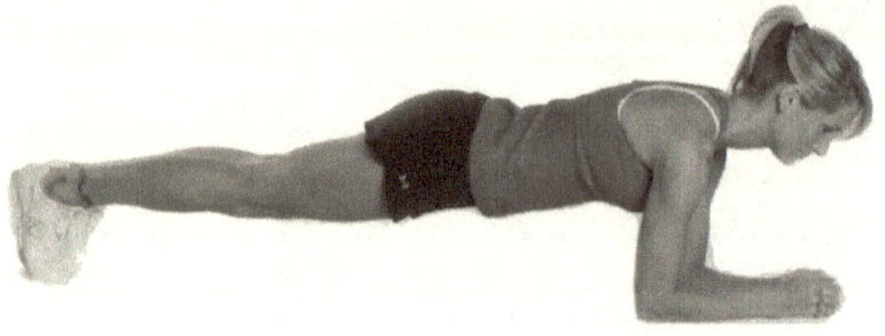

Bear Crawl

Get your hands and knees onto the floor. Lift up your toes, tighten your abs, reach forward with your right arm and knee then do the same with your left arm and knee.

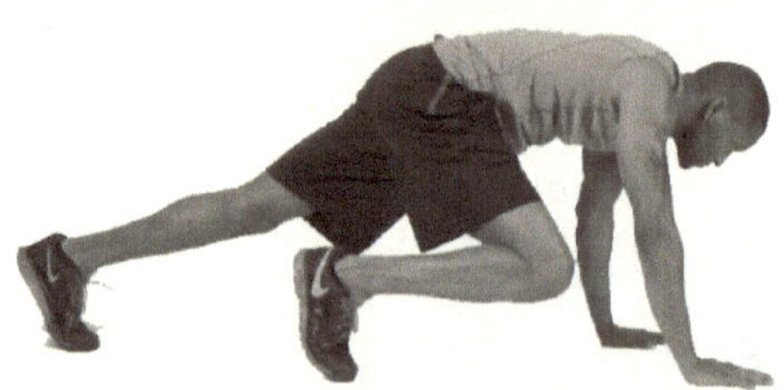

Inchworm

Stand up straight with your feet close together, keep your legs straight and stretch down with your hands on the floor. Start walking your hands forward slowly, alternating with your left and right hands, all while keeping your legs straight and only slightly bending your hips. Keep this up until your body is parallel to the ground in a push up position. Once you' re at a push up position take shorts steps with your feet, continue walking until your feet are close to your hands.

Mountain Climber

Start in a plank position, but with your hands on the floor instead of your forearms. Keep your abs tight, your body straight and shoulders away from your ears. Bring your right knee into your chest then quickly switch and bring your left knee into your chest while putting your right knee back. Continue while alternating knees.

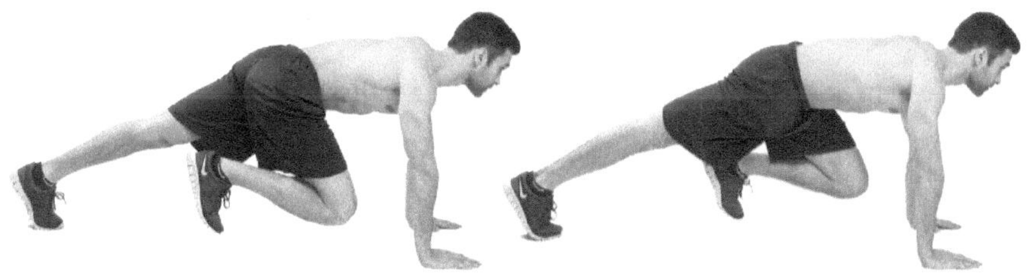

Stair Climb

Walk up and down the stairs while doing biceps curls with a dumbbell or other heavy household object.

Tuck Jump

Stand up straight with your knees slightly bent, then jump as high as you possibly can while bringing your knees towards your chest and arms extended out. Upon landing with your knees slightly bent, jump again.

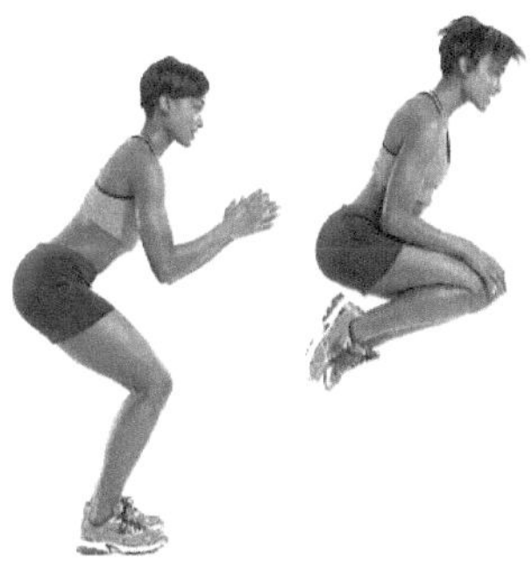

Plank to Push Up

Start in the plank position with your forearms on the floor, keep your body straight and abs tight. Place your right hand on the floor, followed by your left hand. Once you have both hands on the floor you are in a push up position. Perform a push up then return back to the plank position. Repeat while alternating the arm that makes the first move.

Burpees

Crouch down and place your hands on the ground while putting your weight into your arms. Jump and extend your legs. Now with your legs extended, and hands on the floor, keep your elbows tight and close to your torso. Lower yourself with your arms then push yourself up again and jump to go back into the crouching position you started with then stand up. Repeat the process and try to do it as fast as possible.

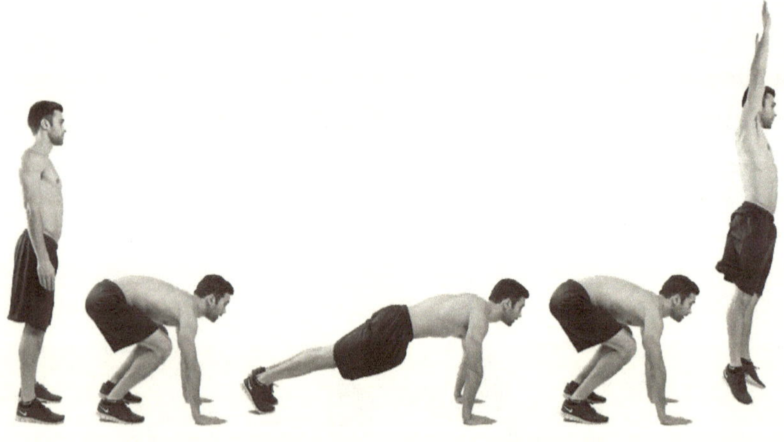

Prone Walkout

Start on all fours and abs tight, then slowly start walking your hands forward while keeping the toes stationary. Once you have reached as far as possible slowly walk the hands back to the starting position all while keeping your abs tight.

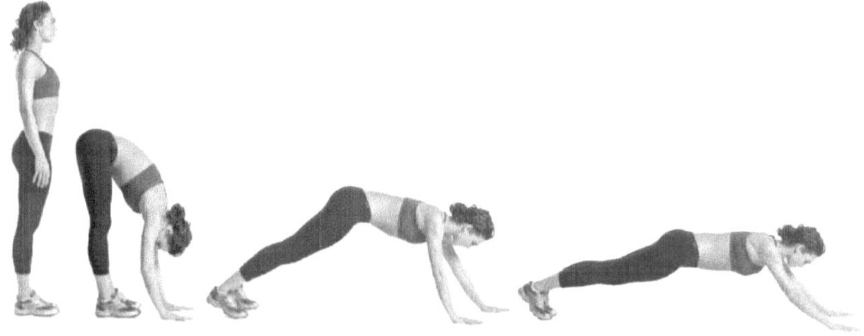

Leg Workouts

Squat

Stand up straight with your feet shoulder width apart and your toes facing forward. Slowly start to crouch by bending your knees and hips until your thighs are parallel to the ground while ensuring you do not lift your heels off the ground. Now press through the heels to return to a standing position.

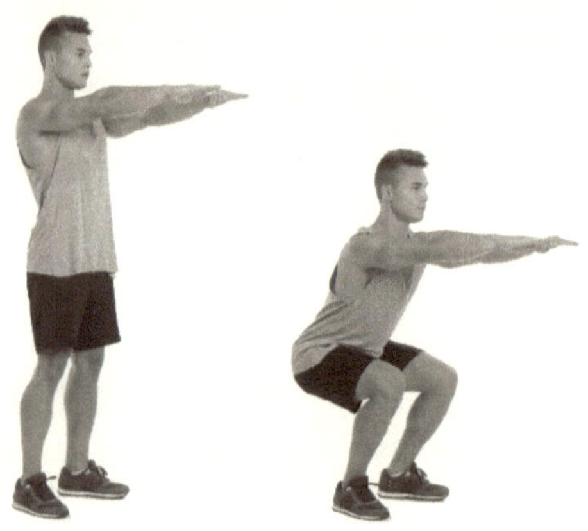

Pistol Squat

Stand up straight and lift one leg off the floor while looking directly forward with your chest up, knees bent slightly and arms pointing forward. This is your starting position. Crouch down into a squat by flexing your hips and knee. While slowly descending, extend your lifted leg to allow enough space for your squat. Hold the squat position briefly, then return back to the starting position by pushing through your heel.

Squat Reach Jump

Same routine as a normal squat, but this time instead of pushing yourself into a standing position push yourself through your heels into a jump with your arms overhead.

Chair Pose Squat

Stand up with your back straight and your feet shoulder width apart. Squat down until your thighs are parallel to the floor while you swing your arms up into the air. Then bring yourself back up by straightening your legs, then lift your right knee up while swinging your left arm outside the right knee. Return back to the starting position and repeat with the opposite leg.

Lunge

Stand up with your back straight, hands on your hips and feet shoulder width apart. Step forward with your right leg and slowly lower your body until your left knee is close to the floor. Slowly return to the starting position and repeat with the other leg.

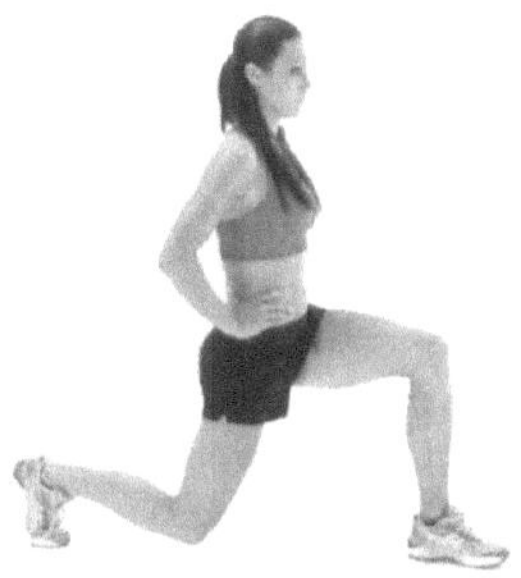

Lunge-to-Row

Start my performing a normal lunge, but this time instead of bringing the forward leg back to the starting position, raise it above the ground while bringing your arms overhead, ensuring your leg remains bent at a 90-degree angle.

Clock Lunge

Stand up with your back straight, hands on your hips and feet shoulder width apart. Step forward with your right leg and slowly lower your body until your left knee is close to the floor. Slowly return to the starting position then take a big step to the right and lunge again. Step back to the centre and lunge back with your right leg.

Lunge Jump

Stand up with your back straight and feet shoulder width apart.
Lunge forward with your right foot, then jump up and bring your
arms straight forward while keeping your elbows bent. While mid-
air, switch legs and land with your left leg lunged forward. Repeat
and alternate your legs.

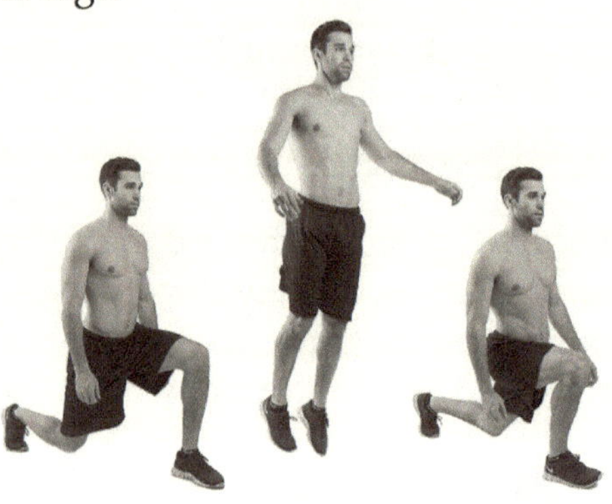

Curtsy Lunge

Stand up straight with your feet side by side and shoulders back.
When lunging, instead of lunging forward, step your left leg back so
that its behind your right leg and to the side. Drop down slowly
ensuring equal weight on both feet and torso is upright. Press back
up and repeat with the opposite leg

Wall Sit

Slide your back down a wall until your thighs are parallel to the
ground or until it looks like you're sitting on an invisible chair.
Ensure your back is straight and your knees are located directly
above your ankle.

Quadruped Leg Lift

Get down onto your hands and knees with your palms shoulder
width apart. Tense your core and raise your right leg up behind you
until it is in line with your torso. Keep your back straight and hold
the position for 5-10 seconds until you lower your leg back down.
Repeat with the opposite leg.

Calf Raises

Stand up and slowly raise your heels off the ground so that you're standing on your toes. Keep your knees straight and hold this position for 2 seconds then slowly come back down until your heels are back to touching the floor. To get a wider range of motion it is a good idea to try this exercise while standing on something elevated.

Step Up

Find something that's elevated from the floor, such as a step or bench. Place your right foot onto the elevated surface and step up until your right leg is straight. Return back to the starting position and repeat with the opposite leg.

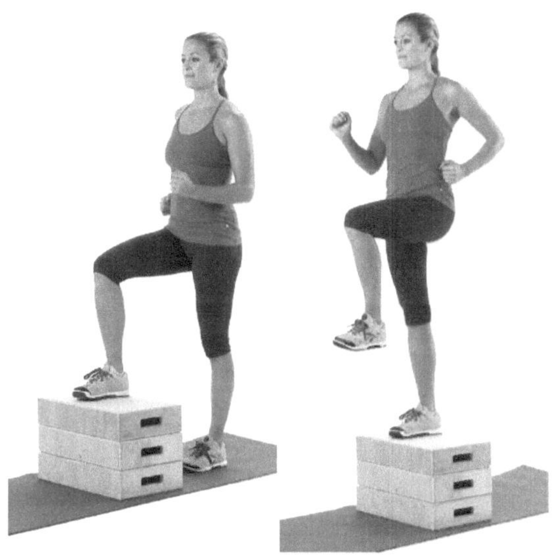

Shoulder and Arm Workouts

Arms Circles

Stand up straight and extend your arms to the sides, making a T shape. With both arms, slowly make clockwise circles for 20 - 30 seconds. Then reverse, making anti-clockwise circles.

Boxer

Start with your feet shoulder width apart, knees bent and torso parallel to the ground. Keep your elbows tight to your waist and hands close to your chest. Extend your left arm forward and your right arm back. Then with both arms extended, bring them back in and repeat, alternating between arms.

Triceps Dips

Seat yourself with your back near a bench or step and knees slightly bent. Grab the edge of the step with your hands a little more than hip-width apart and perform a dip. Straighten your arms back to starting position and repeat

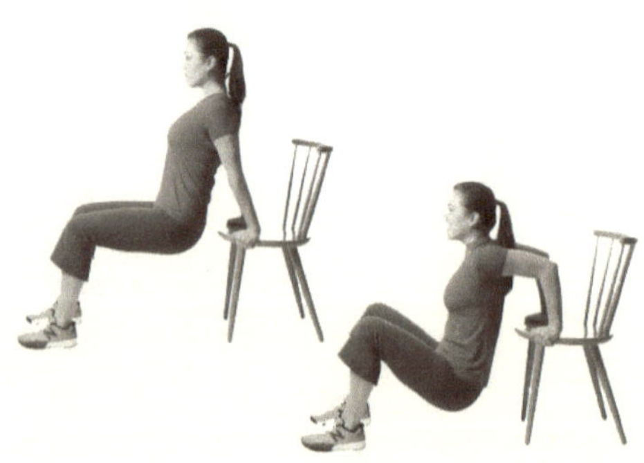

Diamond Push-Up

Get on all fours with your hands together and under your chest. Position your hands so that they make a diamond shape with your index fingers and thumb touching. Elevate your body by extending your arms. Ensure your body forms a straight line from your feet to your head. Lower yourself, making sure that your elbows are not pointing outwards. Stop when your chest is just barely touching the floor, then elevate yourself back to the starting position.

Shoulder Stability Series

Lie down on your stomach, extend your arms overhead with your palm facing each other. Once you're in position, move your arms so that they resemble the following letters. I, Y, T, W, O.

Chest and Back Workouts

Push up

Kneel down onto your knees and bring your feet together behind you. Place your palms flat on the ground, positioning your hands shoulder-width apart. Slowly lower your body by bending your elbows, do not allow your lower back to sag. Continue to lower yourself until your chest or chin touch the floor, then push upwards through your arms, continue this until your arms are fully extended.

Dolphin Push Up

Start with a yoga dolphin pose so that your body resembled an upside-down V shape with your forearms flat on the floor. Lower your shoulders until your head is over your hands, then pull up your arms to return to the starting position.

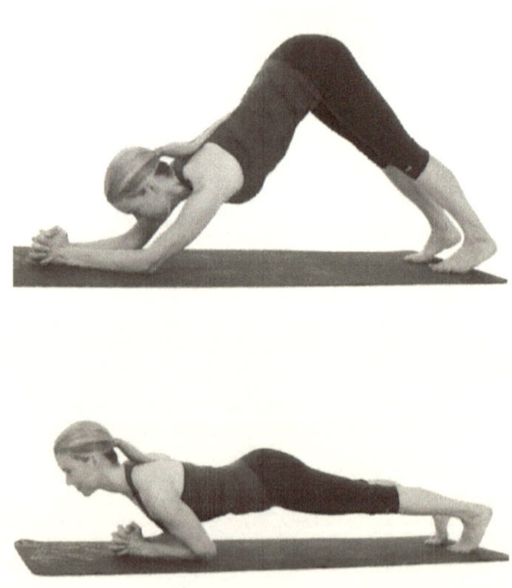

Handstand Push up

Get into a headstand against a wall, make sure your elbows are at a 90-degree angle. Slowly lower your body until your head touches the ground, then lift yourself back up. Ask a friend of assistance in necessary.

Judo Push up

Start off in a push up position but with your hips extend high up. Lower the front half of your body until your chin is barely touching the floor, then move your head and shoulders upwards and lower your hips while keeping the knees off the ground. Do this in reverse to return back to the starting position.

Superman

Lie down on your stomach with your arms and legs extended. Keep your torso stationary while raising the arms and legs so that it looks like you're flying like superman. Hold this position for a few seconds.

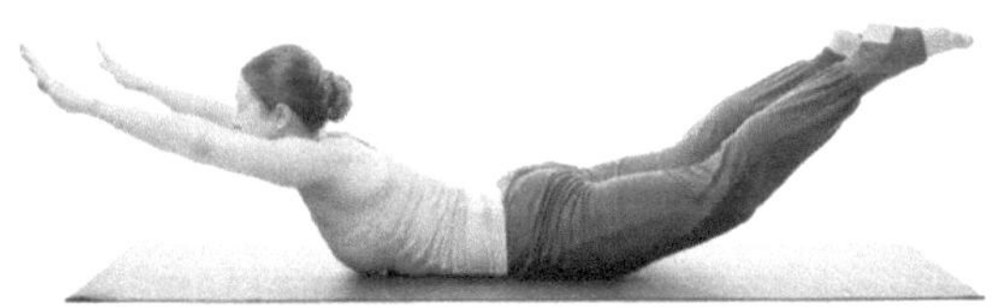

Reverse Fly

Grab two moderately heavy objects such as two bottles of water. Stand up with one foot in front of the other and front knee slightly bent. Face your palms together, tighten your abs and bend forward a little from the waist. Extend your arms out to the side while squeezing the shoulder blades.

Donkey Kick

Start in a push up position with legs close together. Tense your core and kick both legs into the air with knees bent. Try landing gently to avoid injury.

Contralateral Limb Raises

Lie down onto your stomach with your arms stretched and palms facing each other. Slowly lift an arm an inch away from the floor, keeping it straight. Ensure the head and torso stay stationary. Hold your arm at this position for a few seconds before lowering it back down. Repeat and alternate arms.

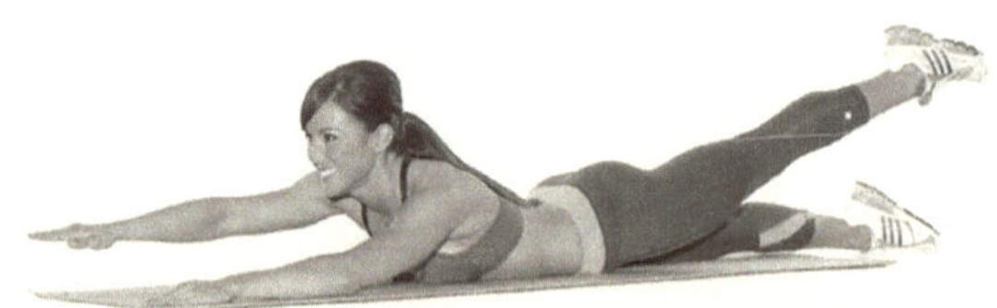

Core Workouts

Flutter Kick

Lay down on your back with your arms to the side and palms facing down. Lift your heels off of the floor and make quick up, down motions with your legs while keeping your abs engaged.

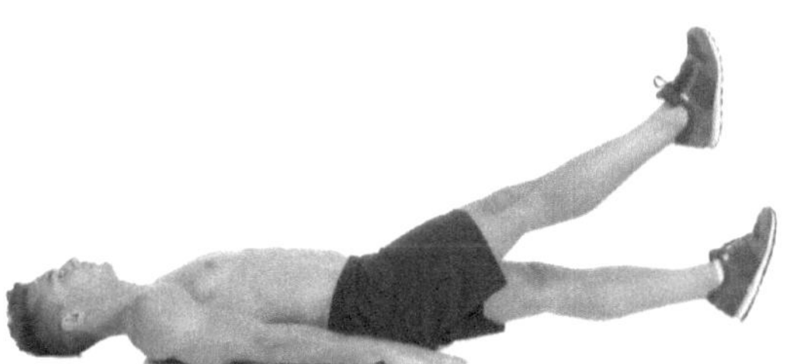

L Seat

Sit down on the floor with legs extended, hands on the floor and arms fully extended. Lift your leg up until it is parallel to the floor. Hold this position.

Side Plank

Lie down to your side, keeping your arm at a 90-degree angle. Lift yourself up while resting on your forearm and activating your core. Point your other arm straight up while also bringing your hip up. Hold this position for 30 - 60 seconds.

Crunch

Lie down on your back with your knees bent and feet on the floor. Move your hands behind your head and tilt your head slightly down. Lift up your head and shoulders by engaging your core. Continue curling up until your upper back is off the floor. Hold this position briefly then lower your head and shoulder slowly back onto the floor.

Bicycle

Lie down on your back with your knees bent and hands behind your head. Tuck your right knee in towards your chest and bring left elbow towards the right knee. Repeat while alternating sides.

Rotational Push Up

After doing a standard push up, rotate the torso to the right and bring your right hand overhead. Return to the starting position and repeat while alternating sides.

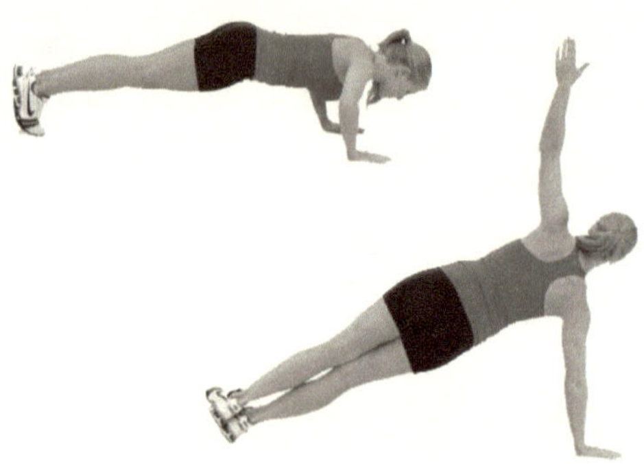

Segmental Rotation

Lie down on your back with your knees bent, arms straight to the side and palms faced towards the ground. Raise up your legs with your knees bent 90 degrees. Slowly rotate the knees as far as you can to the left then hold for 5 seconds. Return the knees back to the middle and do the same towards the right.

Single Leg Abdominal Press

Lie down on your back with your knees bent. Activate your abs by raising your right leg while your knee and leg are bent at a 90-degree angle. Place your right hand on top of your right knee using your core, hold this position for a few seconds before lowering your knee back down. Repeat while alternating sides.

Double Leg Abdominal Press

Same routine as a single leg abdominal press, but instead of lifting up one knee at a time you will lift up both legs while pushing your hands against both knees

Dynamic Plank

Start with a standard plank position with your forearms. Slowly push your hips up, squeezing your abs and hold that position briefly then slowly lower your hips to return back to the plank position.

Russian Twist

Sit on the floor with your legs at a 90-degree angle. Tilt backwards until your feet are lifted a couple inches off the floor. Your feet should be 45 degrees from the floor. Clasp your hands together and twist your torso left and right, activating your core while keeping your head stationary and neck neutral.

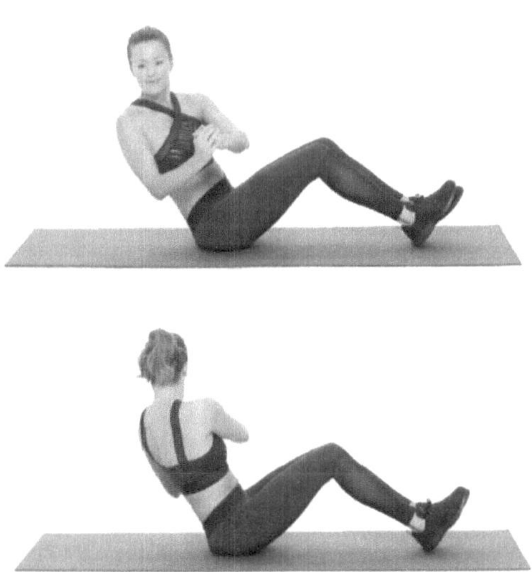

Shoulder Bridge

Lie down on your back with your knees bent and hip distance apart. Lay your arms beside you with your palms facing the floor. Lift up your hips into a bridge position so that your knees, hips and collarbone form a straight line. Bend your right knee towards your chest, then extend your right leg so that your foot is pointing towards the ceiling. Flex your heel and lower your right leg down so that your right knee is parallel to your left knee. Point your right foot and lift your right leg back up, keep doing this for roughly 10 reps then switch legs.

Sprinter Sit Up

Lie down on your back with your arms by your side and legs straight. Bend your elbows at a 90-degree angle and sit up while bringing your left knee towards your right elbow, making them touch. Sit back down and repeat while alternating sides.

30 Day Workout Routine

<u>Day 1</u>
3 Sets Each:

10 Push Up
50 Crunches
20 Squats

<u>Day 2</u>
3 Sets Each:

2 Minutes Plank
2 Minutes Wall Sit

<u>Day 3</u>
5 Sets Each:

10 Push Ups
10 Tuck Jumps
10 Lunge

<u>Day 4</u>
5 Sets Each:

10 Crunches
10 Bicycle
10 Superman

Day 5
4 Sets Each:

10 Rotational Push Up
10 Squats
10 Push Ups
10 Squat Reach Jump

Day 6
3 Sets Each:

10 Mountain Climbers
10 Lunge to Row
10 Calf Raises

Day 7
3 Sets Each:

10 Push Up
20 Crunches
20 Squats
20 Lunges

Day 8

10 Minute Run
10 Push Ups
15 Squats

Day 9
5 Sets Each:

10 Russian Twists
10 Clock Lunges
10 Flutter Kicks

Day 10
4 Sets Each:

20 Crunches
20 Squats
20 Push Ups

Day 11
3 Sets Each:

1 Minute Plank
30 Second Side Plank
1 Minute Plank
30 Second Side Plank

Day 12
3 Sets Each:

10 Seconds Tuck Jumps
30 Seconds Burpees
30 Seconds Mountain Climber
10 Seconds Push Up
10 Seconds Squat Reach Jump

<u>Day 13</u>
4 Sets Each:

12 Lunges
15 Russian Twists
20 Push Ups
15 Squats

<u>Day 14</u>
4 Sets Each (Not Including Run):

1 Mile Run
15 Push Up
20 Crunches

<u>Day 15</u>
5 Sets Each:

15 Mountain Climbers
15 Crunches
15 Push Ups
15 Squats

<u>Day 16</u>
4 Sets Each:

20 Tuck Jumps
20 Crunches
20 Squats
20 Mountain Climbers
20 Push Ups

<u>Day 17</u>
4 Sets Each:

15 Squats
15 Crunches
10 Push Ups
15 Mountain Climbers

<u>Day 18</u>
4 Sets Each:

20 Mountain Climbers
10 Slow Push Ups

<u>Day 19</u>
4 Sets Each:

15 Seconds Push Ups
15 Seconds Tuck Jumps
20 Second Lunge
20 Second Plank
30 Second Mountain Climbers
20 Second Squat Reach Jump

Day 20

10 Minute Run
15 Push Ups
15 Squats

Day 21
4 Sets Each:

20 Seconds Mountain Climber
20 Seconds Push Up
20 Seconds Tuck Jumps
20 Seconds Lunges
20 Seconds Squat
20 Seconds Bicycle

Day 22
5 Sets Each:

10 Russian Twist
10 Crunches
10 Lunge Jumps

Day 23
5 Sets Each:

5 Tuck Jumps
5 Push Ups
5 Crunches
5 Calf Raises
5 Squats
5 Mountain Climbers

<u>**Day 24**</u>
4 Sets Each:

15 Bicycle
15 Push Ups
15 Squats

<u>**Day 25**</u>
3 Sets Each:

10 Squats
20 Crunches
20 Lunges
20 Push Ups

<u>**Day 26**</u>
3 Sets Each:

60 Second Burpees
30 Second Plank
60 Second Burpees
30 Second Plank

<u>**Day 27**</u>
5 Sets Each (Not Including Run):

10 Minute Run
10 Push Ups
15 Squats

<u>**Day 28**</u>
4 Sets Each:

10 Tuck Jumps
10 Push Ups
10 Crunches
10 Bicycle
10 Lunges
10 Second Side Plank

<u>**Day 29**</u>
6 Sets Each:

15 Second Tuck Jumps
15 Second Push Ups
20 Second Squat Reach Jump
20 Second Mountain Climbers
30 Second Crunches
30 Second Calf Raises
20 Second Lunges

<u>**Day 30**</u>
5 Sets Each:

10 Tuck Jumps
10 Segmental Rotation
10 Lunges
10 Squats
10 Crunches

Thank you for taking the time to read this book. Feel free to modify the 30-day routine to fit your lifestyle. Remember good things in life do not come easy, which is especially true when it comes to fitness. I hope I've helped you reach at least one step closer to your goal and wish you the best for your future endeavours.

www.ingramcontent.com/pod-product-compliance
Lightning Source LLC
Chambersburg PA
CBHW051406250726
48656CB00006B/2293